The Search for New Vaccines

[redacted]

The Search for New Vaccines

The Effects of the Vaccines for Children Program

Henry G. Grabowski and
John M. Vernon

The AEI Press

Publisher for the American Enterprise Institute
WASHINGTON, D.C.
1997

We are grateful to a number of individuals who gave us helpful comments and data inputs on this project. They include Morris Friedman, Marge Mitchell, Mark Sanyour, Jeff Tarlowe, and Tom Vernon at Merck; Allison Johnson and Bob Snyder at the Centers for Disease Control; Elaine Esber at the FDA; Jeff Totten of Mercer Management Consulting; Cyndee Long, Marily Ruhdy, and Ron Saldarini at Wyeth-Ayerst; and Leighton Read at Aviron. The opinions and conclusions in this book are our own, as are any remaining errors or omissions.

Available in the United States from the AEI Press, c/o Publisher Resources, Inc., 1224 Heil Quaker Blvd., P.O. Box 7001, La Vergne, TN 37086-7001. Distributed outside the United States by arrangement with Eurospan, 3 Henrietta Street, London WC2E 8LU England.

Library of Congress Cataloging-in-Publication Data

Grabowski, Henry G.

The search for new vaccines : the effects of the Vaccines for Children Program / Henry Grabowski and John Vernon.

p. cm.

Includes bibliographical references.

ISBN 0-8447-4033-0 (paper)

1. Vaccines for Children (Program)—United States. 2. Vaccination of children—Government policy—United States. 3. Immunization of children—Government policy—United States. I. Vernon, John Mitcham, 1937– . II. Title.

RJ240.G73 1997

615'.372'0830973—dc21 97-30439

CIP

THE AEI PRESS
Publisher for the American Enterprise Institute
1150 17th Street, N.W., Washington, D.C. 20036

Printed in the United States of America

Contents

LIST OF TABLES

LIST OF FIGURES

1
The U.S. Vaccine Industry

The focus of this study is on the incentives to invest in R&D for new and improved vaccines in the United States, particularly with regard to the potential effect of the Vaccines for Children program (VFC) on R&D incentives. It is useful to begin with a brief discussion of the nature of the vaccine market, the emergence of the VFC program, and other important industry developments.

The Demand for Vaccines

The 1992 worldwide vaccine market generated sales of approximately $2.7 billion, according to a report prepared for the Department of Health and Human Services (HHS) by the Mercer Management Consulting Company.[1] In terms of worldwide sales, vaccines are a relatively small component of the pharmaceutical market of about $200 billion. Of the $2.7 billion in sales, adult vaccines account for about $620 million, with the remainder being vaccines for children. Mercer's report for HHS subdivided the pediatric vaccines into two categories. First, there are the "basic" vaccines: measles-mumps-rubella (MMR), diphtheria-tetanus-pertussis (DTP), polio, bacille Calmette-Guerin (BCG, the tuberculosis vaccine), and tetanus toxoid (TT). These were developed more than twenty years ago and are now commodities with sales of about $1 billion. Second are the "new" vaccines: haemophilus influenza b (Hib, the meningitis vaccine), hepatitis B (Hep B), hepatitis A (Hep A), and varicella, with about the same number of sales.

While vaccines are a small part of the pharmaceutical market, they have been experiencing rapid growth during the 1990s. One industry source estimated that the global vaccine market had increased to $3.3 billion in 1995 (a more than 20 percent advance over 1992 sales).[2] A key driving force in this market expansion has been the growth of the new pediatric vaccines. The acellular pertussis vaccine and the varicella vaccine were introduced into the U.S. market and were important factors in the global market expansion of vaccines since 1992.

Because of licensing requirements, the U.S. vaccine market can be viewed as separate from that of the remainder of the world.[3] To market vaccines in the United States, companies must be licensed by the Food and Drug Administration (FDA). Unlike the requirements in many other countries, the FDA requires both a product and an establishment license. In 1993 only seven firms were licensed by the FDA to supply all the childhood vaccines. The market for individual vaccines is also highly concentrated, but there are prospective new entrants from the biotech sectors. These issues are discussed further in the next section.

An important economic factor on the demand side of the U.S. pediatric vaccine market is the role of government as a major purchaser. Vaccines are purchased by the government at prices much below those paid by the private sector. These "public" prices are negotiated on an annual basis with a federal agency, the National Centers for Disease Control and Prevention (CDC). The "private" price is that set by manufacturers for private-sector buyers. To illustrate, table 1–1 lists the prices for the years 1985–1996 for three important vaccines: DTP, MMR, and OPV (oral polio). In 1996, for example, the ratios of the public-to-private prices for the three vaccines were 25 percent, 54 percent, and 20 percent, respectively.[4]

Table 1–2 shows the percentages of total vaccine dosages purchased by the government for 1985–1995. The share of government purchases increased from about a

TABLE 1–1
PRIVATE CATALOG PRICES AND FEDERAL CONTRACT PRICES PER DOSE FOR CHILDREN'S VACCINES, 1985–1996
(dollars)

	DTP[a]		*MMR*[b]		*OPV*[c]	
Year	*Private*	*Public*	*Private*	*Public*	*Private*	*Public*
1985	2.80	2.21	13.53	6.85	6.15	0.80
1986	11.40	3.01	15.15	8.47	8.67	1.56
1987	8.92	7.69	17.88	10.67	8.07	1.36
1988	6.47	3.90	19.67	11.74	7.78	1.07
1989	6.09	3.40	19.67	11.74	9.16	1.63
1990	6.09	2.35	19.63	10.27	9.45	1.63
1991	5.41	1.70	20.85	10.89	9.16	1.71
1992	5.48	1.44	20.85	10.89	9.62	1.80
1993	5.38	1.43	20.85	10.89	10.14	1.87
1994	5.54	1.33	20.85	11.22	10.18	1.92
1995	5.54	1.40	21.43	11.27	10.18	1.92
1996	5.54	1.40	22.12	11.87	10.18	2.03

NOTES: Prices exclude the excise taxes for the Vaccine Injury Compensation Program instituted in 1988. The excise taxes are $4.56 per dose of DTP, $4.44 per dose of MMR, and $0.29 per dose of OPV. These taxes were suspended on December 31, 1992, and reinstated on August 10, 1993.
a. DTP is diphtheria-tetanus-pertussis vaccine.
b. MMR is measles-mumps-rubella vaccine.
c. OPV is oral polio vaccine.
SOURCE: National Centers for Disease Control and Prevention, Atlanta, 1997.

third of the market in the mid-1980s to roughly half the market in the early 1990s. Another major increase in the percentages purchased by the government is now taking place as a result of the Vaccines for Children program. The VFC program was enacted in 1993 and first implemented in the last quarter of 1994. As shown in table 1–2, government shares in the vaccine market actually declined during the transition year of 1994. In 1995, however, the first

TABLE 1–2
PUBLICLY PURCHASED DOSES OF CHILDREN'S VACCINES AS A PERCENTAGE OF NET DOSES DISTRIBUTED IN THE UNITED STATES, 1985–1995
(percent)

Year	*DTP*[a]	*MMR*[b]	*OPV*[c]
1985	15	38	32
1986	29	44	39
1987	45	51	46
1988	33	47	44
1989	35	50	44
1990	40	45	48
1991	43	52	52
1992	48	55	50
1993	49	46	54
1994	37	44	48
1995	56	69	63

a. DTP is diphtheria-tetanus-pertussis vaccine.
b. MMR is measles-mumps-rubella vaccine.
c. OPV is oral polio vaccine.
SOURCE: Division of Immunization, National Centers for Disease Control and Prevention, Atlanta, 1997.

full year of the VFC program, a significant expansion in government shares occurred compared with pre-VFC levels. Preliminary data indicate that this growth continued in 1996.[5] Although there is uncertainty about what the equilibrium government share will be under the VFC program, the CDC has estimated that an increase to about 80 percent of the market is possible.[6]

Background of the VFC Program

A number of government programs made vaccines free to children prior to the VFC program.[7] These programs were Medicaid, section 317 of the Public Health Services Act of

1962, and the initiatives of various states. Of course, Medicaid covers children from families with incomes near the poverty level. The section 317 program enabled any child to receive the federally contracted vaccines free of charge at a public health clinic. Before the VFC program began, twelve states combined Medicaid, section 317 funding, and state funds to offer free vaccine to all providers for all patients in their practices, including those who are fully insured.[8]

In early 1993, the Clinton administration announced a plan "under which the Federal Government and the states would buy up all childhood vaccines, then distribute them free to public clinics and private doctors' offices to make sure that all children are properly vaccinated."[9] The Clinton plan was based on a belief that "only 40 percent to 60 percent of preschool children get the recommended shots" and that the high cost of vaccines was a major factor in this low rate of vaccination. Both the percentages used by the Clinton administration and the cost barrier hypothesis have been disputed as being incorrect. For example, Robert Goldberg argues, using HHS data, that the correct immunization rate for children was near 90 percent, not the 55 percent figure used by HHS Secretary Donna Shalala.[10] Correspondingly, a General Accounting Office (GAO) report concurred with this finding and also concluded that "the cost to parents of vaccines has not been a major barrier to children's timely immunization."[11] Nevertheless, significant elements of the Clinton plan were enacted into law.

Section 13631 of the Omnibus Budget Reconciliation Act of 1993 (OBRA, 1993) created the VFC, to begin by October 1, 1994. The VFC is an entitlement program for four groups of children through eighteen years of age. The first three comprise those eligible for Medicaid, those who are American Indians, and those who are medically uninsured. The fourth group, children who have medical insurance that does not cover childhood vaccinations—the "underinsured"—are eligible for VFC vaccines but may receive them only in federally qualified health centers or rural health clinics. In addition to the three vaccines charted in tables 1–1 and 1–2, the VFC also covers hepatitis B (Hep B), the haemophilus influenza type b (Hib), and varicella (chicken pox) vaccine. The varicella vaccine was approved for marketing by the FDA in 1995, and the VFC program approved its coverage, with some restrictions by age cohort, in 1996.

The main coverage change embodied in the VFC program is the ability of uninsured children to obtain free vaccines from any enrolled private practitioner rather than having to obtain them from public health clinics. Another potentially significant effect comes from the encouragement of additional universal-purchase states. The VFC program gives the states the right to purchase vaccines for non-VFC eligible children at CDC contract prices. By the end of 1996, three additional states had elected universal purchase status, and several others had extended benefits to part of the non-VFC eligible population.[12] The contract prices of established children's vaccines (MMR, DTP, and oral polio [OPV]) are capped at 1993 levels under the legislation, subject to an annual adjustment for inflation.

As mentioned above, the intended goal of the VFC program is to increase children's immunizations. It operates under the premise that price and convenient access are the chief barriers to immunization. A number of studies on compliance, however, indicate that factors such as parental awareness, education, and a dysfunctional medical delivery system for poor children are the primary barriers to immunizations.[13] The VFC program is targeted to vaccine purchases, not to programs that address these barriers in populations with low vaccination rates. Furthermore, it is likely to result in substitution effects that are questionable on policy grounds—namely, the federal purchase of vaccines at controlled prices for individuals who are not poor and who have vaccine coverage through the private sector. Such substitution effects will be especially significant if several more states elect to become universal-purchase states under the VFC program.

Clearly, a major increase in government purchases from 50 percent to possibly 80 percent at below market prices will result in reduced cash flows for the vaccine firms and increased uncertainty concerning the returns to new vaccine introductions. This can be expected to lead to lower R&D spending and, as a result, fewer new and improved vaccines. This unintended side effect of the VFC program is a major theme of this study, and we will report our econometric analysis of the effect later.

Important Industry Developments and Characteristics

The vaccine industry in the United States is highly concentrated. The number of firms licensed by the FDA to manufacture vaccines has declined from twenty-six in 1967 to seventeen in 1993, with the greatest decline occurring between 1967 and 1980. In the case of the pediatric market, eleven firms were producing childhood vaccines in 1980, and this number fell to seven by 1993. The seven suppliers consisted of three domestic companies, two state laboratories, and two foreign-owned firms.[14] There was a sole-source manufacturer for ten of the fifteen childhood vaccines. In terms of individual vaccines, Connaught has more than 50 percent of the DTP market, with Lederle having 25–33 percent. Merck has all of the MMR market and Lederle has all of the oral polio market.

In 1985, the Institute of Medicine (IOM) issued a study on vaccine supply and innovation.[15] At that time, the industry was besieged with a number of adverse trends that are chronicled in the IOM study. In particular, beginning in the mid-1970s, several major pharmaceutical firms decided to exit the vaccine business. During the same period, the proportion of total pharmaceutical R&D devoted to biologicals and vaccines also declined significantly.

Among the major factors cited for this exodus from the vaccine business were the increased number of liability suits filed against manufacturers, increased regulation and rising R&D costs, and lower risk-adjusted expected returns for vaccines as compared with other pharmaceutical businesses. The situation in vaccines posed a major public policy dilemma, given that vaccines have assumed a major role in the reduction and even eradication of several significant infectious diseases. Indeed, cost-benefit analysis of the development of the polio vaccine shows social benefits exceeding costs by a factor of more than 10 to 1.[16] Several other vaccines also demonstrated very favorable benefit-cost ratios in studies by economists.[17]

Fortunately, the situation in vaccines is much more promising today than it was a decade ago. There has been a renaissance in terms of innovative effort. New and improved vaccines, including combinations, have been introduced over the past decade for haemophilus influenza type b, hepatitis A and B, varicella, and pertussis. There have been large investments in vaccine R&D by the biotech industry, using the tools of molecular biology. The major suppliers have also significantly increased their vaccine R&D, including many collaborative programs with smaller biotech firms.[18] As we discuss in the next section, there is currently an impressive pipeline of R&D projects involving new vaccines for a number of major pediatric and adult diseases.

One important development that improved prospects for this industry was a change in the product liability situation. Vaccines may be associated with certain adverse effects, most often in the form of mild reactions, but in extremely rare circumstances they may cause life-threatening conditions and death. While the benefits of approved vaccines exceed the risks by large margins, the number of product liability cases filed against manufacturers increased substantially in the early 1980s, as several courts moved to a strict liability standard. For example, lawsuits against DTP manufacturers increased from four in 1980 to 255 in 1986. Increased product liability costs were a major factor underlying the rapidly rising prices and falling number of U.S. vaccine suppliers during this period.

In 1986, Congress passed the National Childhood Vaccine Injury Compensation Act in an attempt to stem these trends. The act provides no fault compensation to persons injured by a vaccine for certain childhood diseases. Prospective cases are paid out of the Vaccine Injury Compensation Trust Fund, which is funded by excise taxes on covered vaccines. Excise taxes per dosage are $4.56 for DTP, $4.44 for MMR, and $0.29 for polio. The act has reduced vaccine liability costs and reduced the number of liability cases, and this contributed to a more favorable economic environment for vaccines.

Another positive development for vaccines was the rapid growth of managed care and integrated health care delivery systems during the 1990s. The traditional fee-for-service health care insurance system favored diagnostic and therapeutic technologies, as compared with preventive technologies. Given responsibility for the total health care costs of patients, integrated managed care systems have greater incentives to be concerned with both preventive and treatment technologies. The coverage of the recently introduced varicella vaccines by several of the large managed care groups illustrates this increased sensitivity to the benefits of preventive approaches.

Given these various developments, it is instructive to consider the long-term trend of R&D investment in vaccine R&D by pharmaceutical firms. Figure 1–1 shows the percentage of total R&D that is allocated to the biologicals by member firms of Pharmaceutical Research and Manufacturers of America (PhRMA). While biologicals include products in addition to vaccines, vaccines account for most of the R&D in this class.[19]

The figure shows the decline in the percentage of pharmaceutical R&D devoted to biologicals, from more than 5 percent in the early 1970s to just over 2 percent in the early 1980s. Following the passage of the 1986 act and other positive developments discussed above, there was a strong upswing in the percentage of R&D devoted to biologicals

FIGURE 1–1
BIOLOGICAL R&D AS PERCENTAGE OF TOTAL R&D, 1971–1994

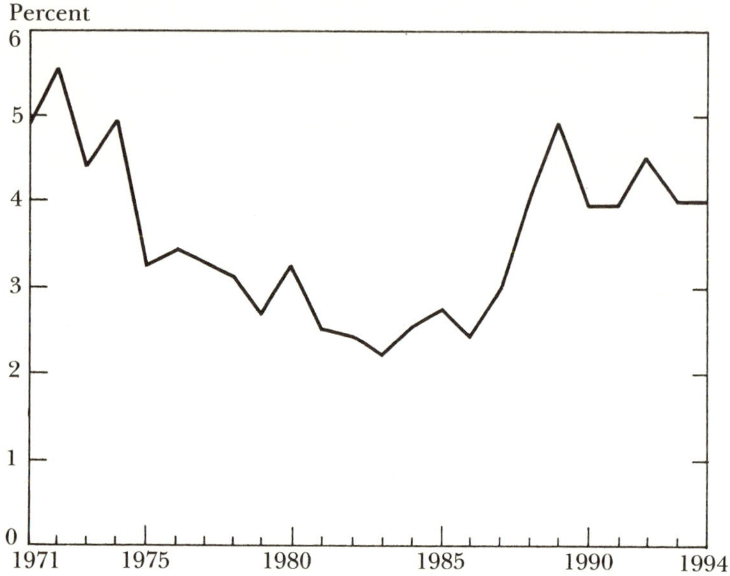

SOURCE: Pharmaceutical Manufacturers Association Annual Survey Reports, 1971–1993; PhRMA Industry Profile, 1996.

and vaccines for a decade. It has averaged more than 4 percent in the 1990s. Furthermore, these data do not capture the substantial vaccine R&D investment in recent years of the expanding biotech sector (since most biotech firms are not members of PhRMA). Investment in vaccine R&D has clearly responded to the more positive economic signals and opportunities surrounding this industry in recent years.

The Potential for Future Advances

During the past decade, there has been a renaissance of interest in developing new vaccines for a number of pediatric and adult diseases. *The Jordan Report,* a semiannual report published by the National Institute of Allergy and Infectious Diseases (NIAD), reflects the great optimism that now exists about scientific progress in vaccines.[20] During 1996, there were 285 vaccine R&D projects in progress (not including HIV vaccine efforts), of which 133 were already in clinical trials. Major targeted disease areas of this research effort include respiratory diseases, viral hepatitis, sexually transmitted diseases, herpes virus diseases, parasitic diseases, and fungal infections.

One of the major sources of this excitement comes from the application of biotechnology to vaccine innovation. Indeed, biotech approaches have been at the forefront of the efforts to develop a new generation of vaccines using genetic engineering techniques. The recombinant vaccines for hepatitis B are illustrative of this approach. Currently, recombinant vaccines are in clinical development for several major diseases, including herpes simplex, Lyme disease, and colon and breast cancer.[21]

Research efforts are now moving toward "DNA vaccines," a "third"-generation technology that injects genes into the body to produce foreign proteins that induce powerful immune system defenses.[22] This approach is targeted to major diseases such as influenza, tuberculosis, AIDS, cancer, and malaria. The tests in animal models have been very promising, and human trials are underway. DNA gene vaccine R&D is being performed by biotech firms such as Apollon and Vical, as well as major vaccine companies such as Merck and American Home Products. Other biotech firms, such as Auragen and Chiron, are also pursuing this approach, and the National Institutes of Health (NIH) is participating in joint research ventures with several firms.

While there is great excitement about the prospects for major scientific advances in vaccines, the process of developing a new vaccine involves a long and costly investment process. This process includes large-scale clinical testing and FDA approval. The relevant economic factors are discussed in detail in the next section. If a program like VFC significantly lowers the available funds for and expected returns to new pediatric vaccines, one can expect a shift in R&D investments from pediatric vaccines to adult vaccines, as well as to other pharmaceutical and nonpharmaceutical projects.

Biotech R&D projects are especially vulnerable to government policies that change the returns to R&D. Biotech firms typically focus on the early, risky stages of R&D in the hopes of inventing new technology or products that can be licensed to large global suppliers, who can provide the necessary capital and market access for commercialization. Most biotech firms are small, with little cash flow, and they rely importantly on venture capital, initial public offerings, and partnerships with larger firms. As the chief executive officer of one such company, Aviron, said in congressional testimony: "Biotechnology investors who support the early stage of vaccine innovation are exquisitely sensitive to the economic signals being sent from Washington."[23]

2
Economics of Vaccine Innovation

A major interest in this book is to trace the likely effect of changes in public policy regarding government purchases of vaccines for children on future vaccine innovation. Since investments in vaccine R&D are business decisions, it is natural to begin with the determinants of R&D profitability. In this regard, investments in vaccine R&D, as in the case of other investment decisions, will be driven by considerations of expected returns relative to the costs of investment funds.

Determinants of R&D Returns

We will outline briefly the key parameters and variables that influence the returns to R&D in the broader pharmaceutical industry. The vaccine industry is a part of this industry—though with some important differentiating characteristics, considered in further detail below. In this section, we analyze the key economic factors that affect the returns to pharmaceutical and vaccine R&D investments. In identifying these factors we rely on a recent study that we performed on the profitability of all new chemical entities (NCEs) introduced in the U.S. pharmaceutical industry over the 1980–1984 period.[1] In subsequent sections, we consider how vaccine R&D investment decisions are differentiated from pharmaceuticals.

To illustrate the important elements of R&D investment

decisions, we present in figure 2–1 a cash-flow diagram for the average NCE introduced in the United States in the 1980–1984 period. Clearly, there is a long period of negative cash flows—some fourteen years. These negative cash flows are followed by a comparable period of positive cash flows. The cash-flow values over the lifetime of a project, as shown in figure 2–1, determine the internal rate of return (IRR), a key measure of the financial merit of an R&D project.

The long period of negative cash flows reflects two types of costs: R&D costs and plant capital costs. The R&D costs begin in year −11 in figure 2–1, with preclinical discovery costs. (Note that the R&D costs include costs allocated for drugs that never make it to market, and there are clearly many "dry holes" in the discovery phase.) Another five or six years of negative cash flows reflect the clinical testing phases, followed by several years of waiting for FDA approval before marketing can begin. The large dip in the negative cash flows at year −1 is attributable to the construction costs of plant and equipment for manufacturing the new drug. This construction, of course, must be completed prior to the initiation of marketing of the NCE in year 1.

A major difference between pharmaceuticals and vaccines discussed below is the timing of the plant investment. In vaccines the plant must be completed much earlier than in pharmaceuticals in order to obtain an establishment license from the FDA—a requirement unique to vaccines and biologic products. Because of the time value of money, the earlier investment for an equivalently valued plant tends to lower the internal rate of return.

The life cycle of revenues that begins in year 1 in figure 2–1 and lasts for twenty years is, obviously, a key determinant of positive cash flows. Also important is the contribution margin, or the proportion of revenues that represents profits and the contribution to R&D investment. The particular pattern of revenues is influenced greatly by the existence of substitute products (branded or generics) at different stages of the life cycle. For example, upon patent

FIGURE 2–1
CASH FLOWS FOR REPRESENTATIVE NEW CHEMICAL ENTITY
INTRODUCED BETWEEN 1980 AND 1984
(millions of $1990)

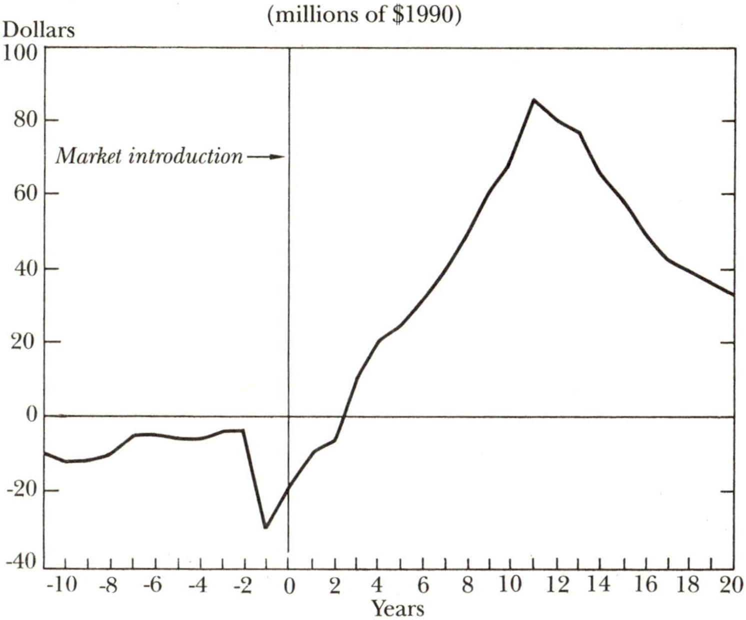

SOURCE: Henry Grabowski and John Vernon, "Returns to R&D on New Drug Introductions in the 1980s," *Journal of Health Economics,* November 1994.

expiration—shortly after the peak in figure 2–1—generics have been winning progressively larger shares of the brand name product's market.

While generic competition has not been an important factor in vaccines as it has in pharmaceuticals, the margin is particularly important in vaccines because of current policy issues regarding government purchases at prices lower than those paid by private purchasers. The margin, of course, is related to the price-cost difference. Clearly, a shift toward more government purchases will tend to lower the average margin in vaccines—and, therefore, the profitability of vaccine R&D investment.

In the remainder of this chapter, we consider differences between vaccines and drugs with regard to the various determinants of the economics of innovation. These factors include R&D costs, plant costs, the life cycle of revenues, and the contribution margin. While there are considerably fewer data available for vaccines than for pharmaceuticals, they indicate some important differences between these two product categories.

R&D Costs

The vaccine R&D process is similar to that for drugs in that there is a period of basic research or discovery followed by the filing of an investigational new drug (IND) application with the FDA, and then a period of clinical trials. During the phase III clinical trials (or after their completion), the manufacturer files a product license application (PLA) and establishment license application (ELA) with the FDA. The period between the first submission of the PLA and the ELA and the final approval by the FDA usually takes about two years or longer.[2] Therapeutic pharmaceuticals, unlike vaccines, are not required to obtain the ELA—they submit a new drug application (NDA) only, which is similar to the PLA.

In May 1996, the FDA issued a final rule in which it relaxed the ELA requirement for some well characterized biotechnology products, but it continued to hold vaccines to the dual licensing requirement. "FDA disagrees that vaccines . . . should be included within the scope of this rule at this time because these products raise additional concerns in assessing safety, purity, and potency. For vaccines, safety is a critical concern due to the intended use in a healthy population."[3] Hence, a key difference between vaccines and drugs is the requirement that vaccines must have their plants licensed. We will return to this issue shortly in the discussion of plant costs.

While there are no public studies of vaccine R&D costs

as there are for drugs, a 1985 Institute of Medicine study is instructive in this regard. The object of the study was to set priorities for important disease targets for which it was judged technically feasible to develop new or improved vaccines within a decade's time. The IOM committee that performed this study included experts from academia, government, and industry. As part of its analyses, the IOM committee developed estimates on the probabilities of technical success, incremental development costs, and time periods for licensure for several candidate vaccines. In undertaking this task, the IOM committee interacted with a broad spectrum of outside consultants that were knowledgeable concerning the economics of the vaccine development process.

The IOM analysis is not based on a representative sample of vaccines. Indeed, only vaccines that had at least a 50 percent predicted chance of technical success within a ten-year horizon were included in the committee's analysis. Hence, it does not provide representative information on success probabilities. The IOM study does, however, provide estimates by experts on expected development costs for vaccines that can be compared with survey data analyses of new drug development costs. In table 2–1, we have reproduced the committee's estimates on incremental development costs and times for eight pediatric-related vaccines that were not yet in clinical testing in the United States in 1985. (Vaccines such as varicella and hepatitis B, which were already in clinical testing in 1985, are excluded from table 2–1 because the committee's incremental estimates would underestimate clinical development costs and times.)

It is instructive to compare the estimates on these IOM-predicted development costs and times with those of the DiMasi et al. study, which investigated R&D costs for a sample of new chemical entities first tested on humans in the 1970–1982 period.[4] In the DiMasi study, the mean out-of-pocket clinical costs for successful NCEs was $32 million ($1987). This corresponds to predicted development costs

TABLE 2–1
INSTITUTE OF MEDICINE ESTIMATES OF DEVELOPMENT COSTS AND TIMES FOR PEDIATRIC-RELATED VACCINES, 1985

			Development to Licensure		
Pathogen	*Vaccine Envisaged*	*Target Population*	Probability of technical success, %	Estimated future costs, $millions	Time to licensure, years
Bordetella pertussis	Acellular	Infants	0.90	20	3–5
Cytomegalovirus	Glycoprotein produced by recombinant DNA technology	All children	0.50	45	7–10
Hepatitis A virus	Subunit	Susceptibles of all ages (routine for children)	0.95	25	5
Herpes simplex viruses 1 & 2	Attenuated live virus	Children up to age 12 and older susceptibles	0.50	30	8

	Glycoprotein produced by recombinant DNA technology	Children up to age 12 and older susceptible	.090	30	5
Neisseria gonorrhoeae	A small number of promising options need investigation to determine best approach	Adolescents and adults age 15 and over	0.50	50	10
Parainfluenza viruses	Trivalent, subunit vaccine (must contain fusion protein)	Infants	0.80	25	5
Respiratory syncytial virus	Glycoprotein produced by recombinant DNA technology; attenuated live virus	Infants	0.80	25	5
Rotavirus	Attenuated live human or reassortment virus	Infants	0.90	20	2–4

SOURCE: Institute of Medicine, *New Vaccine Development, Establishing Priorities,* vol. I (Washington, D.C.: National Academy Press, 1985), chapter V and related appendixes.

of $20–50 million for the eight vaccines from the IOM study in table 2–1. Although the two studies are very different in scope, it would appear that the expected out-of-pocket clinical testing costs for new vaccines are comparable in magnitude to those of new chemical entities.

Of course, the total expected costs of discovering and developing a new drug or vaccine will include not only the expenditures for successful entities but also the expenditures for product candidates that fail. In the case of pharmaceuticals, the clinical success rate was 23 percent, so that the costs of failed compounds were substantial. Another major element of R&D costs involves the research or discovery stage. The DiMasi et al. study estimated the out-of-pocket R&D costs (in $1987) for the representative new drug introduction to be $115 million (including both the discovery and clinical testing phase and incorporating the costs of failures). Furthermore, the DiMasi study capitalized these expenditures to the date of marketing, to take account of the implicit interest or time costs associated with the lengthy R&D period. This resulted in a capitalized cost of $231 million ($1987) to discover and develop a new drug entity.[5]

Although very little systematic information is available on these other factors influencing total R&D costs, there are some indications that the probability of success is higher and development times are lower for vaccines. A 1989 paper by Hardegree et al. cited a 33 percent clinical success rate for vaccines, but it did not specify what data it used to obtain this value.[6] A success rate of 33 percent would be at the upper range observed for different therapeutic classes in pharmaceuticals. It would be comparable in value to the clinical success rates observed for anti-infectives (30.2 percent), the pharmaceutical category with the highest success rate.[7]

Clinical development times have averaged 8.3 years for recent NCE introductions.[8] This involves approximately 6.0 years in clinical testing and 2.3 years for FDA approval.

There is considerable variability associated with different therapeutic classes and other factors. The estimates in table 2–1 on the expected time to licensure for new vaccines range from four to ten years. These estimates suggest somewhat faster development periods than have been the case in pharmaceuticals.

Table 2–2 shows the FDA approval times for important pediatric vaccines introduced since 1986 (hepatitis B, Hib, acellular pertussis, and varicella). The FDA review time ranges from eighteen months to fifty-five months for the first introduction of these vaccines. This is not dissimilar to the experiences of new chemical entities, which have averaged about thirty months of FDA review time (with a wide variance around this mean). The introduction of user fees has resulted in faster review times since 1994 for new chemical entities. The review times of vaccines may also benefit in the future from user fees.

Biopharmaceutical Approaches to Vaccine Development

Since vaccines are increasingly produced using biotechnology, one might gain some knowledge of expected vaccine success rates and times by examining the experience of biopharmaceutical products. Two initial studies of success rates for biotech drugs were performed by Bienz-Tadmor et al.[9] and Struck.[10] Both studies found that success rates for biotech drugs were substantially higher than success rates for NCEs discussed above. In particular, both studies projected success rates for biopharmaceuticals in excess of 50 percent. A basic assumption implicit in the methodology of these studies, however, is that success rates for biotech drugs that entered development in the late 1980s and early 1990s are the same as for the biotech drugs that entered development in the early- to mid-1980s. This is a strong, and potentially erroneous, assumption, given that 90 percent of drugs in their samples were still under active testing.

TABLE 2–2
FDA REVIEW TIME FOR IMPORTANT PEDIATRIC VACCINES AGAINST
HEPATITIS B, HIB, ACELLULAR PERTUSSIS, AND VARICELLA, 1986–1995

Vaccine and Diseases It Immunizes Against	*Company*	*FDA Review Time (months)*	*FDA Approval*
Recombivax® HB Hepatitis B Vaccine, Recombinant	Merck, Sharp and Dohme	18	7/1986
ProHIBIT® Haemophilus b Conjugate Diphtheria Toxoid Conjugate	Connaught Laboratories, Inc.	55.4	12/1987
HibTITER® Haemophilus b, Conjugate Diphtheria, CRM 197 Protein Conjugate	Praxis Biologics, Inc. (Owned by Lederle Laboratories)	22.5	12/1988
Engerix-B® Hepatitis B Vaccine, Recombinant	SmithKline Biologicals	20.8	8/1989
PedvaxHIB® Haemophilus b, Conjugate Vaccine	Merck, Sharp and Dohme	24.9	12/1989

Haemophilus influenzae type b conjugate vaccine (infant indication)	Praxis Biologics, Inc.	6.9	10/ 1990
Haemophilus influenzae type b conjugate vaccine (infant indication)	Merck	4.1	12/1990
ACEL-IMUNE® Acellular Pertussis DTP	Lederle-Praxis Biologicals	51.5	12/1991
Tripedia™ Acellular Pertussis DTP	Connaught Laboratories, Inc.	27.1	8/1992
ActHIB™ *Haemophilus influenzae* type b conjugate vaccine, tetanus toxoid conjugate	Pasteur Merieux Serums et Vaccins	27.8	3/1993
TETRAMUNE™ DTP and *Haemophilus influenzae* type b conjugate vaccine (infant indication)	Lederle-Praxis Biologicals	14.9	3/1993
Varivax chicken pox	Merck	26	3/1995

SOURCES: FDC Reports, "The Pink Sheet," March 20, 1995; M. Sing and M. K. Willian, "Supplying Vaccines: An Overview of Market and Regulatory Context." In M. Pauly, ed., *Supplying Vaccines: An Economic Analysis of Critical Issues* (IOS Press, 1996).

Recently, Gosse et al. analyzed a comprehensive sample of U.S. biopharmaceutical drugs and compared the success rates between older and newer biotech entities.[11] They found dramatic differences in the time pattern observed for early versus later biotech drug cohorts. Although new biotech drugs still have success rates somewhat higher than do new drugs, the success-rate curve for recent cohorts more closely resembles that of new chemical entities rather than that of early biological entities.

The first biological entities introduced into the market were naturally occurring proteins that replaced purified nonrecombinant formulations already in general use as established therapies (for example, insulin and human growth hormone). Similarly, the first recombinant vaccine for hepatitis B supplanted a plasma-derived vaccine. It is reasonable to expect that recombinant versions of established therapies would have high success rates, once the technology to manufacture these products was proven. Other, earlier targets for biotechnology were naturally occurring proteins with well-known and defined physiologic activity (erythropoietin). As the biotech drugs move to targets in which limited knowledge exists about clinical and pharmacological profiles, it is reasonable to expect that success rates would fall back toward those of conventional drug entities. This is consistent with the findings of the recent Gosse et al. study.

It is not clear at this point how recombinant-produced vaccines fit in the evolving picture for biotech drugs more generally. As discussed in the first section, the scientific knowledge base appears to be very strong, and there is currently great optimism about the possibility of developing vaccines for a number of major disease areas using biotech approaches.[12] On this basis, it is reasonable to postulate that vaccines have above-average *expected* probabilities of success as compared with NCEs. It is still very early, however, to evaluate actual success rates for vaccines using recombinant techniques, and the data for doing so are not publicly available at this time.

The performance of biotech products with respect to development times is still evolving, but it parallels the experience observed with success rates. In particular, the earliest biotech drug introductions had much shorter average development times than new chemical entities had. But clinical development times of recent biopharmaceutical introductions have been increasing.[13] The sample of new biologic entities that have been introduced in the marketplace is still very small (twenty-nine products between 1980 and 1994), and the variance in clinical development times by indication and other characteristics is very large. For example, new recombinant entries involving immunologic indications had an average clinical development time of 86.7 months, while those involving the endocrine system (insulin and human growth hormones) had an average clinical time of 35 months.

In sum, there is some basis for expecting that recombinant vaccines are characterized by higher success rates and faster development times as compared with new chemical entities. Quantifying this expectation and evaluating the implications for capitalized R&D costs, however, require more data and further research. Furthermore, the advantages that vaccines may enjoy in this regard are likely to be offset, partly or entirely, by greater pre-market capital outlays as compared with new chemical entities. This issue is discussed in the next section.

Plant Costs

As noted above, vaccines require both a product license and an establishment license from the FDA's Center for Biologics Evaluation and Research (CBER). The application for the establishment license, the ELA, describes the facilities, equipment, and personnel involved in the manu-

TABLE 2–3
FDA PRODUCT AND PROCESS REQUIREMENTS,
PHARMACEUTICALS VERSUS BIOLOGICALS

Area	*Pharmaceuticals*	*Biologicals*
Product definition	Product defined by: certificate of analysis	Product defined by: process; process controls; facility; facility practices; certificate of analysis
Product license	Yes	Yes
FDA batch release	Not typical	Typical
Process specs	General	Detailed
Facility license	No (Drug Master File used)	Yes (Establishment License Application)
Focus	Finished drug	Bulk drug substance
Multiproduct facility	Common	Uncommon

SOURCE: Authors, based on interviews with government and industry officials.

facturing process. Vaccine manufacturers also have to satisfy the FDA that they have followed establishment licensing standards and current Good Manufacturing Practices, an extensive body of regulations for manufacturing pharmaceuticals and biologicals.[14]

The differences in product and process requirements for biologicals and pharmaceuticals are summarized in table 2–3. CBER still requires individual production batch release for every vaccine product made or sold in the United States. By comparison, pharmaceuticals are typically licensed via the NDA and then sold based on a certificate of analysis. One consequence of the rigid production processes imposed by CBER is that they keep vaccine manufacturers from enjoying the cost reductions gained by learning curve benefits and continuous process improvements. Pharmaceutical production processes are upgraded regularly to yield cost savings. Furthermore, vaccines are seldom produced in a multiproduct facility as are pharmaceuticals, and it is difficult and expensive to convert biological facilities to other uses.

Because of the complexity of scaling up pilot production of vaccines to production at commercial levels, the FDA also "strongly encourages manufacturers to produce clinical materials for phase III studies in a commercial production facility."[15] This introduces another major difference between vaccines and drugs, since a commercial plant must be built for phase III trials of vaccines (table 2–4), but not for drugs. (As noted above, certain well-characterized biological products no longer face this requirement, as a result of a 1996 rule change.)

Dr. Lance Gordon, CEO of a small biotechnology company, OraVax, testified in 1995 congressional hearings regarding his disagreement with this FDA policy. "An important corollary of the establishment license requirement is the policy that Phase III clinical trials done to obtain marketing approval must be done in the establishment to be licensed. This has required companies such as Zoma, Synergen, Repligen and many others to invest in commercial production facilities, often over $30 million in construction costs alone, prior to knowing if their products would work in the clinic."[16] Dr. Gordon argued that a better approach would be to follow the approach used for other pharmaceutical products—that is, to require only a product license.

Hence, a clear difference in the economics of vaccine

TABLE 2–4
MANUFACTURING BY PHASE,
PHARMACEUTICALS VERSUS BIOLOGICALS

Production Phase	*Pharmaceuticals*	*Biologicals*
Phase I/II	Lab or pilot	Pilot facility
Phase III	Pilot facility	Commercial facility
Commercial	Commercial facility	Commercial facility

SOURCE: Authors, based on interviews with government and industry officials.

and drug innovation turns on the need to establish manufacturing capacity in vaccines several years in advance of product approval. Even for plants of the same dollar value, the fact that vaccine plants are required a number of years earlier in the investment process makes for much higher capitalized plant costs for vaccines. Bader has investigated the extra costs for biotech products attributable to the requirement that an operational plant be in place prior to phase III testing (a five-year lead time in his analysis).[17] He found that the extra interest and operational costs cause the capitalized investment requirements of a minimum $25 million scale plant to more than double. These findings demonstrate the significant extra cost burden imposed on biological and biopharmaceutical manufacturers by these CBER requirements.

Vaccines also generally involve a more capital-intensive production process than do chemical drug entities, because of higher sterilization requirements and a more involved system of process controls. A recent study prepared for the U.S. Agency for International Development by Lederle-Praxis Biologicals is instructive in this regard.[18] The study estimated the cost of constructing a large-scale manufacturing facility for DPT and polio vaccine in Russia that could meet U.S. quality standards and produce up to 30 million doses per year of these vaccines. The facility relied on external sources to supply the concentrates and performed only the bulk batching, filling, and packaging of the vaccines. The estimated cost for this facility in Russia was $103 million, which is comparable in value to what it would cost in the United States.[19] The high capital intensity of vaccine production is also reflected by the fact that Merck and Co. recently spent $150 million to construct a biotechnology facility for vaccines in West Point, Pennsylvania.[20]

The large capital investment requirements in vaccines have constituted one of the major factors contributing to the high concentration of vaccine suppliers discussed earlier. Of course, a new entrant can start with a small-scale plant, but this subjects the firm to the higher production costs associated with suboptimal scale plants, as well as the high regulatory costs of altering or switching facilities when demand reaches capacity levels.

Product Life Cycle of Revenues

The patterns of revenues for vaccines and for therapeutic pharmaceuticals have rather different underlying forces. For example, if one focuses on pediatric vaccines, the market is "as predictable as it is limited. The size of the market is defined by the birth cohort in the United States, roughly 4 million live births annually, and the number of visits children make to clinics or pediatricians to receive necessary booster shots."[21]

A recent study computed the compound annual rate of growth of total doses for the three older pediatric vaccines for the period 1982–1993.[22] The growth rate was basically flat for OPV and DTP. MMR grew at 11 percent, but this was attributable to a second-dose recommendation for MMR during the period, which increased the number of doses in a predictable manner.

Pharmaceutical revenues, conversely, follow a pattern that is roughly captured by figure 2–1, which shows cash flows after market introduction. Cash flows, of course, are revenues minus cash outlays, so the pattern of revenues can be inferred as rising for ten to twelve years, followed by a period of decline. Obviously many factors are important—the incidence of disease, competitive drugs, and pricing strategies.

The declining phase for drug revenues has been greatly affected in recent years by generic competition at the time of patent expiration. In other studies, we have found that leading pioneer drugs, on average, lose more than 50 percent of their revenues in the first year after patent expiration.[23] The amount of revenue erosion is much larger for some recent expirations of large-selling pharmaceuticals like Tagamet.

The effects of patent expiration and generic penetration in vaccines have so far been quite different. With regard to the older vaccines, patents are apparently unimportant. According to industry sources, MMR is produced by a single supplier in the United States because of that supplier's superior product, and OPV has a single supplier because of the FDA's reluctance to license other firms.

Generally, vaccines have been perceived to be more difficult to patent than drugs—given the fact that vaccines are natural substances. Nonetheless, this perception has been changing in the wake of advances in biotechnology, and the courts recently have shown a willingness to grant patents for some natural substances. This is the case, for example, where the substance can be produced through recombinant techniques in large quantities and high degrees of purity.

The hepatitis B vaccine is a good example. Hep B has fourteen different patents and a number of organizations with royalty rights. According to one study, "because so many organizations own royalty rights to Hep B, its royalty payments approximate 13 to 15 percent of sales. Hib and DTaP royalties are more typical, at 4–6 percent of sales."[24]

TABLE 2–5
COMPARISON OF MARGINS AND COSTS OF VACCINES AND PHARMACEUTICALS BY PERCENTAGE OF SALES

	Vaccine Industry	*Pharmaceutical Industry*
Margin	44	46
S,G, and *A*	24	35
COGS	32	19
Total	100	100

NOTES: Margin is contribution to R&D, interest, taxes, and earnings. *S, G,* and *A* is selling, general, and administrative expenses. *COGS* is cost of goods sold.
SOURCE: Mercer Management Consulting, *Report on the United States Vaccine Industry,* Commissioned by the Department of Health and Human Services, June 14, 1995, Exhibit 30, p. 33.

Contribution Margins

The 1995 *Report on the United States Vaccine Industry* by Mercer Management Consulting contains a useful comparison of the average costs and contribution margins of vaccines and pharmaceuticals. The results are reproduced in table 2–5.

Interestingly, the contribution margins (to R&D, interest, taxes, and earnings) are quite similar—44 percent in vaccines, versus 46 percent in pharmaceuticals. But the cost components vary considerably.

For example, vaccine production requires greater process controls and higher sterilization requirements. "The analogy has been made that pharmaceutical manufacturing is similar to chemistry, whereas vaccine production is more like agriculture: drugs can be synthesized and put in tablet form within days to weeks; however, it can take a year or more, with complicating intervening steps, between the first culture of a vaccine product and its eventual use in a child."[25]

Also, there are higher distribution costs for vaccines. Vaccines are generally shipped through overnight services and must be kept at cold temperatures because of their heat sensitivity. In addition, shipments of a large share of vaccines are sent in small quantities directly to individual physicians—as compared with pharmaceuticals, which are shipped to large pharmaceutical wholesalers. The result is that the cost of goods sold (COGS) for vaccines is 32 percent, versus only 19 percent for pharmaceuticals. (Of the 32 percent COGS in vaccines, distribution costs account for 9 percentage points.)

The other major cost component, selling, general, and administrative (S,G, and A), is 35 percent for pharmaceuticals and only 24 percent for vaccines. The lower selling and promotion costs in vaccines are attributable to the fact that more than half of children's vaccines are sold to the federal and state governments and that children must be immunized to attend school. The number of doctors warranting personal detailing visits is much smaller than for most pharmaceutical products, and therefore sales and promotional expenses for vaccines are relatively low.

The numbers in table 2–5 for vaccines are "blended" values, based on an approximate split with a 50 percent share of unit sales occurring in the public sector and a 50 percent share in the private market. As discussed in our introduction, however, the prices realized in the public sector are dramatically lower than in the private market (table 1–1). This means that profits per unit are much higher on private sales, even after allowing for the lower unit costs for distribution and promotion to the public sector. For example, the Mercer Report estimates that the contribution margin on private sales of MMR and oral polio vaccines is $8.40 per dose versus $2.90 per dose for public sector sales.[26]

It is the private market sales that have provided the dominant share of the firm's return on capital investment and R&D. Furthermore, the private market yields most of the cash flows that established firms utilize to fund R&D for new vaccines, both in house and in collaboration with biotech entities. If the VFC program eliminates most of the remaining private market vaccine purchases, this can be expected to have very adverse consequences for vaccine R&D. Chapter 4 provides some quantitative analysis of this issue, using a model of R&D investment determinants that is estimated on pharmaceutical industry data.

Distribution of Returns

Finally, a very important characteristic of the innovation process that has been ignored thus far should be mentioned. Up to this point, we have been focusing our attention on the factors that determine the mean return to R&D. From the point of view of the individual investor or firm, the *distribution* of returns to NCEs is also meaningful. This point is illustrated in figure 2–2. It portrays the distribution of returns for the sixty-seven NCEs introduced between 1980 and 1984. The measure of financial merit is taken to be the net present value (NPV) of net revenues, and this is compared with the average capitalized value of R&D costs. The drugs are grouped into ten deciles, and it is evident that there is great dispersion of returns.

Figure 2–2 shows that only the top three deciles covered the fully allocated average R&D cost. In fact, the top two deciles—about fourteen drugs—accounted for more than 70 percent of the total present value generated by these sixty-seven NCEs. Even though the majority of the sixty-seven NCEs have present values substantially below the fully allocated R&D cost, it is still true that many of these "unprofitable" drugs do contribute to firm profits. That is, in many cases an unprofitable drug more than covers its own incremental development and capital costs. As

FIGURE 2–2
AFTERTAX PRESENT VALUES BY DECILE FOR NEW CHEMICAL ENTITIES INTRODUCED BETWEEN 1980 AND 1984
(millions of $1990)

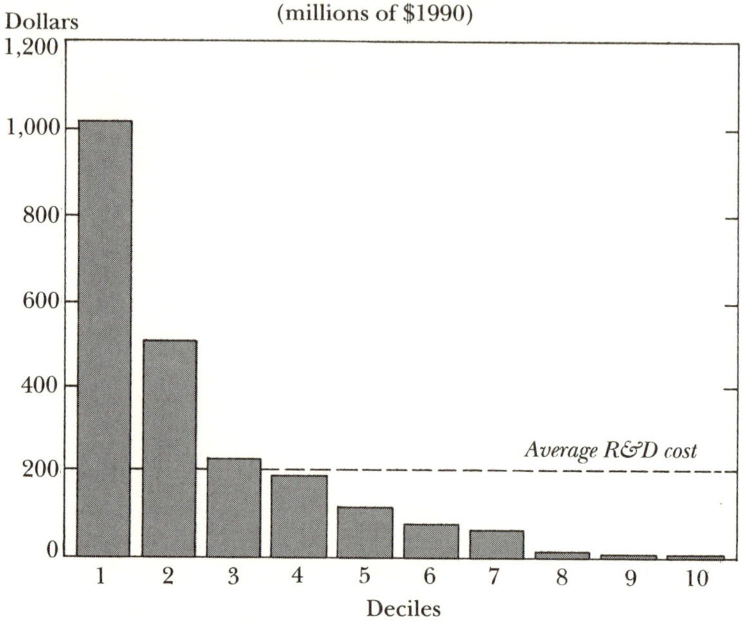

SOURCE: Henry Grabowski and John Vernon, "Returns to R&D on New Drug Introductions in the 1980s," *Journal of Health Economics,* November 1994.

noted earlier, however, the average R&D cost also includes an allocation for drugs that drop out along the development path and are never marketed. Clearly, a particular firm must cover the costs of unsuccessful drug candidates. Hence, with such a skewed distribution, it is critical that a firm have an occasional big winner or a drug in the top two deciles if it is to cover all its R&D costs over the long run.

Because vaccines have been characterized by only a handful of new introductions since the early 1980s, it is difficult to determine whether the underlying distribution of returns is as skewed as in pharmaceuticals. As noted, the market for pediatric vaccines is subject to some limiting demand-side factors that are not present for pharmaceuticals. Correspondingly, however, vaccines like pharmaceuticals are subject to large fixed costs from products that fall by the wayside in the development process. These costs must be covered by the small number of commercially successful introductions if this process is to remain viable over the long run. As the president of Merck's vaccine division has indicated in this regard, "Over the past thirty years Merck has invested more than $1.1 billion in vaccine research, more than half of which was spent investigating products that never made it to the market."[27]

From a strategic perspective, both businesses are being strongly affected in the 1990s by the increased cost consciousness on the part of payors. In particular, as a result of the growth of managed care, pharmaceutical firms are increasingly focusing on the development of unique therapeutic entities that can command a premium price and offer significant value to cost-conscious providers. The renaissance in vaccine innovational activity is being driven in considerable part by similar concerns.

The primary concern of innovators with regard to the VFC program is that after putting several hundred million dollars at risk for a new vaccine, they will have to sell it essentially to one customer and negotiate the price after the product is approved for marketing by the FDA. In this situation, the firm bears the risk while the government retains enormous advantage in terms of its bargaining power, particularly given the fact that the lion's share of the costs to produce the new vaccine has already been incurred in R&D before the bargaining occurs. As the president of Aviron testified before Congress, "As a vaccine innovator with a high degree of confidence that our products will offer value for money, I would prefer to negotiate prices in a marketplace comprised of well-informed managed care buyers than with a dominant government purchaser. The VFC undermines this market."[28]

3

A Conceptual Model of the Effects of the VFC Program on Vaccine R&D

The major economic effects of OBRA and the VFC program on vaccine R&D activities result from the increased federal government contract purchases at capped prices for children's vaccines. While it is uncertain what percentage of vaccines will be purchased through this contractual mechanism, HHS estimated it could be 80 percent or more if several additional states elect universal purchase status. This would be a major change from the recent past, in which approximately half of all children's vaccines were purchased through federal contracts.

From an economic perspective, this expansion in government purchases at reduced prices affects R&D expenditures for future vaccines in two basic ways. First, for established vaccine manufacturers, it reduces the revenues and cash flow generated by existing products and thereby reduces the availability of funds to invest in new vaccines. Second, it negatively affects expectations about the returns on new vaccines.

For existing vaccines, the VFC program caps prices at 1994 levels, plus an annual increase no greater than the consumer price index (CPI). The VFC program does not subject new drugs to immediate price caps. Manufacturers are put in the potential position, however, of negotiating the future prices for new vaccines with the Centers for Disease Control and Prevention as a dominant purchaser. As discussed, the government in this situation would have very strong market power, and average prices for vaccines can be expected to be much lower compared with the mixed public-private market situation that now prevails. Hence, the prospect of a dominant government purchaser of vaccines will negatively affect the expected returns on future vaccines.

From a conceptual standpoint, it is useful to analyze these effects in terms of the standard investment model of the firm. The firm first assesses the expected returns on vaccine R&D projects, including the different risk profiles of alternative investments. It then uses this information to construct a marginal rate of return schedule or demand curve for investment funds. This is shown in figure 3–1. The curve labeled *D* depicts the demand for funds at alternative returns. This curve can be imagined as a ranking of potential investment projects, with the project with the highest return ranked first, the second highest ranked second, and so forth.

Investment in Vaccine R&D

The level of investment in vaccine R&D will also depend on the cost of funds. Recent work on firm investment behavior supports the hypothesis that the cost of internal funds is less than that for new equity financing (and new debt financing).[1] This is shown in figure 3–1 by the horizontal stair-step–like supply function of funds for investment. There are many theoretical reasons given for the indicated difference in the cost of internal and external funds. They include transaction costs, tax advantages, agency problems, costs of financial distress, and asymmetric information. We will not attempt to explain all these reasons here; they have been discussed at length in the literature.

The existence of a cash-flow effect on firm investments depends on the hypothesized difference in internal and

FIGURE 3–2
EXPECTED EFFECTS OF THE VFC PROGRAM ON R&D INVESTMENT

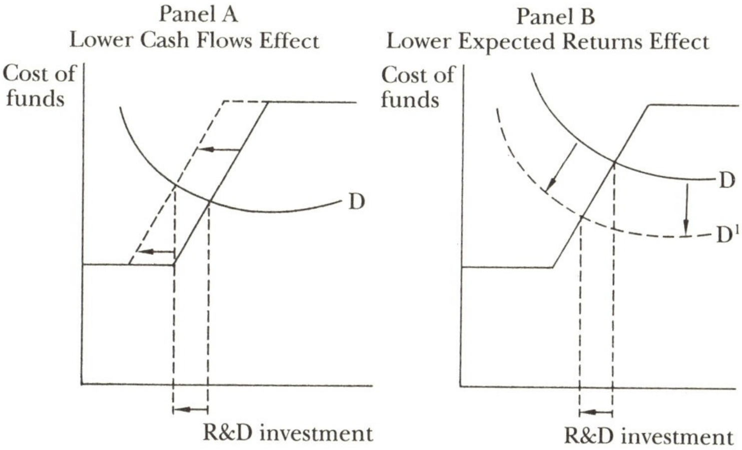

SOURCE: Authors.

vaccine introductions causes the MRR, or *D* curve, to shift to the left (panel B). This also results in a lower reduced level of R&D expenditures.

Of course the size of these negative effects on R&D expenditures is an empirical question. In the remainder of this volume, we consider whether increasing federal purchases to approximately 80 percent under VFC can be expected to have a significant negative effect on R&D expenditures targeted to new vaccines.

For established pharmaceutical firms, vaccines constitute a separate product division that must compete with other product categories for investment resources. For example, figure 1–1 shows that when product liability concerns and other adverse factors negatively affected the expected returns in the 1970s, R&D investment in vaccines declined relative to pharmaceuticals. While there are significant differences between vaccines and pharmaceuticals, which are documented in the last chapter, R&D investment in vaccines and other categories are ultimately governed by the same basic economic forces—namely, expected returns relative to the cost of funds.

The analysis in the next chapter examines R&D investment decisions in vaccines initially from the perspective of the large, established pharmaceutical firms. We then subsequently discuss the situation of the smaller biotech vaccine firms.

FIGURE 3–1
THE R&D INVESTMENT DECISION

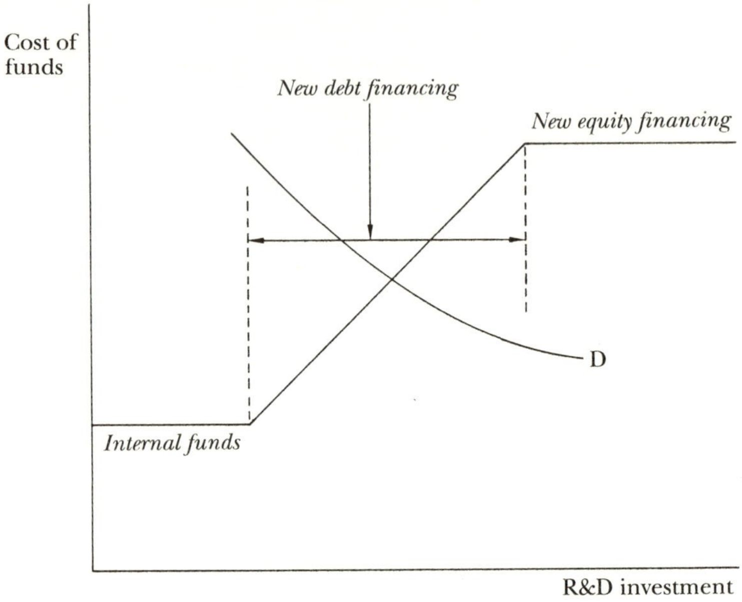

SOURCE: Authors.

external finance. In particular, if there were no differences between the cost of internal and external funds, the level of a firm's cash flow would have no effect on investment decisions. But there is a substantial body of empirical work that supports the existence of a cash-flow effect for U.S. capital investments. In this regard, an earlier study of our own provides strong support for a cash-flow effect for the R&D expenditure of pharmaceutical firms.[2] This is discussed further below.

We can analyze the expected effects of the VFC program in terms of figure 3–2. First, the reduction in cash flow associated with lower revenues from increased government purchases causes the cost of funds to rise and equilibrium R&D investments to decrease (panel A of figure 3–2). Second, the lower expected returns on future new

4

An Empirical Analysis of R&D Determinants

In our earlier study of the 1962–1975 period, we developed and estimated a model of the determinants of firm research intensity: that is, the firm's R&D-sales ratio.[1] The current study makes use of a sample of eleven major pharmaceutical firms over the period 1974–1989.[2]

As in our earlier work, we estimate a model of the following type:

$$R = f\,(IRR,\ Cashfl,\ Pcpharm), \qquad (4\text{–}1)$$

where *R* is a firm's research intensity in a given year, *IRR* is an index of its expected returns from R&D, *Cashfl* is a measure of its cash flow deflated by sales, and *Pcpharm* is the percentage of its total sales accounted for by pharmaceuticals.

It should be noted that the data used to estimate equation 4–1 involve the firm's total R&D outlays, which include expenditures for both pharmaceuticals and vaccines. It is impossible to obtain data separately for vaccine R&D expenditures on an individual firm basis. As discussed above, vaccines are a relatively small component of the total pharmaceutical industry (figure 1–1). Nevertheless, it is reasonable to conclude that vaccine R&D projects will be governed by the same core economic forces as pharmaceutical R&D projects—namely, the size of expected returns relative to cost of funds. This is our basic premise in estimating an

FIGURE 4–1
RATIO OF AGGREGATE R&D TO SALES OF PHARMACEUTICALS, 1974–1989

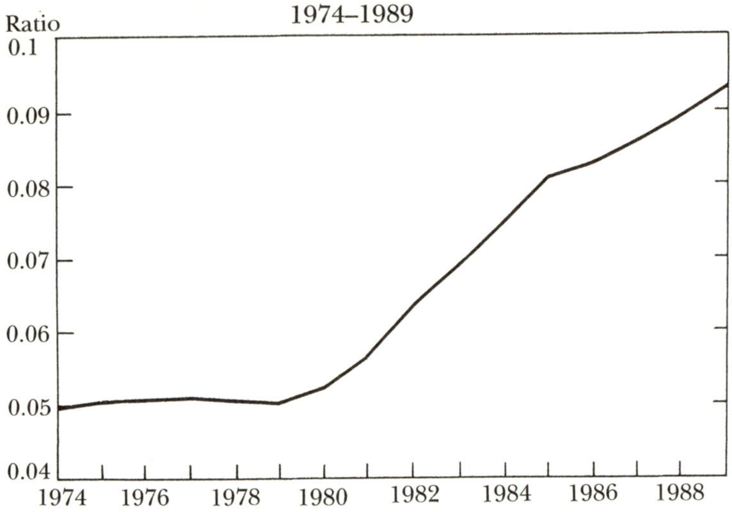

SOURCE: Standard and Poor's Compustat Tape for eleven-firm sample (ref. 51).

aggregate model of R&D determinants that includes both pharmaceuticals and vaccines. The application of this model to analyze VFC intervention effects is discussed further below.

In contrast to the earlier period in which the average R&D-sales ratio for the sample fell over time, in the current period it is generally flat, through about 1978, and then it rises throughout the remainder of the period. This trend is shown in figure 4–1. Despite this significant difference, it is interesting to note that, as we shall explain, our findings for the current period are broadly consistent with the earlier period—namely, that the coefficients of the expected returns and cash flow variable in the regression that explains research intensity are positive and statistically significant.

Data Sample and Explanatory Variables

Data on firm R&D expenditures were obtained from the Standard and Poor Compustat Tape. Two major considerations in selecting the sample of firms to include in the study were the availability of R&D expenditures for the complete 1974–1989 period and a high degree of specialization of the firm in ethical drugs. (As noted, we included the percentage of ethical drug sales to total sales as an explanatory variable in the regressions.)

In addition to the percentage of sales accounted for by pharmaceutical sales—the variable *Pcpharm,* described above—the two major variables are a measure of the expected returns from R&D and the firm's cash-flow variable.

These two variables represent the two factors depicted in figure 3–2. That is, the prospective return to new R&D investment in the figure is represented by how far to the right the *D* curve is. The higher the prospective return, the higher will be the R&D intensity. We use proxy measures to capture this effect, which we will refer to as the demand effect. We use each firm's after-tax cash flow, denoted as *Cashfl,* to capture the second factor, the cash-flow effect.

In our empirical model we tried two alternatives to capture the *IRR,* or the prospective return effect. The first alternative was an index of the industry's recent past success in R&D, as reflected in its sales of new chemical entities per R&D dollar, or *Newsal.* This was similar to the variable employed in our earlier study, except that in that work we used the firm's own past success variable rather than the industry variable. This variable can be criticized on the basis that a firm's prospects for the future may be completely unrelated to its own history.[3] Using the industry variant of this variable, *Newsal* partially corrects for that deficiency.

In fact, the statistical results were quite good for this past success variable. Nevertheless, in view of the obvious difficulty of developing a variable to capture the *prospective* return on R&D investment, we thought it prudent to experiment with an alternative profitability variable as well. In this regard, we decided to use the industry's current profit margin to index expectations. That is, the *Imarg* variable is a weighted average of pre-tax profits as a percentage of sales for the pharmaceutical divisions of the eleven major health-oriented firms.

The *Cashfl* variable was computed as the firm's own profits after taxes, plus depreciation, plus R&D expenditures, divided by sales. To distinguish this variable from current prospects, we lagged the variable two years—as we did in our earlier study.[4]

Empirical Results

The empirical analysis involves estimating various specifications of equation (4–1) on the determinants of research intensity for eleven pharmaceutical firms over the period 1974–1989 (and various subperiods). Detailed empirical results for a number of specifications are presented in the appendix. Since the results are not substantially affected by the choice of functional form, we concentrate here on the findings using the linear functional form.

Table 4–1 provides summary findings for the estimated coefficients and elasticities using the linear regression equation. We provide a range of coefficient estimates given that there are two alternative forms of the IRR index variable (*Newsal* and *Imarg*) and two time periods considered (1974–1989 and 1980–1989). The results are quite strong, and they favor the hypotheses put forth. All coefficients are highly significant and have the expected algebraic signs.

The coefficients of *Cashfl* in the four equations estimated are remarkably close in magnitude, ranging from 0.27 to 0.31. These values are also in the same range as the estimates found in our earlier study, which covered a very different period. Since both the R&D and the cash flow variables in this regression are sales deflated, this coefficient indicates that a $1 loss in cash flow on average results in a $.27 to $.31 decline in R&D.

TABLE 4–1
ESTIMATED COEFFICIENTS AND ELASTICITIES FOR THE EXPECTED RETURNS AND CASH FLOW VARIABLES

Variable	*Coefficients*[a]	*Elasticities*[b]
*IRR*1		
(*Newsal*)	0.17–0.19	0.61–0.70
*IRR*2		
(*Imarg*)	0.62–0.74	1.93–2.55
Cashfl	0.27–0.31	0.77–0.82

NOTES: Based on linear regression of R&D intensity for eleven pharmaceuticals for the periods 1974–1989 and 1980–1989; see table A1.
a. All coefficients are statistically significant at the 1 percent level; see table A1.
b. Elasticities are computed at the sample means; see table A4.
SOURCE: Authors' calculations.

The coefficients of the demand effect variables, *Imarg* and *Newsal*, are also all positive as expected and have high *t*-statistics (they are statistically significant at the 1 percent level). In interpreting the economic significance of these variables, it is especially appropriate to consider their elasticities at the sample mean. The estimated elasticities are quite high, ranging from somewhat below 1.0 in the case of the *Newsal* variable to more than 2.0 for the *Imarg* variable. This indicates that a firm's research intensity in pharmaceuticals is highly sensitive to the expected returns on R&D. This finding is also in accordance with our past research work.

Application to Vaccines

The statistical analysis performed in the previous section pertains to a pharmaceutical firm's total R&D portfolio of projects. Specifically, this analysis indicates that a firm's total R&D intensity is sensitive to expected returns to R&D and to the availability of cash flow. It is reasonable to expect that these aggregate findings also apply in a decentralized fashion to separate business decisions operating within the firm—that is, to vaccines, pharmaceuticals, medical devices, and so forth. The past trends in vaccine R&D allocation to biologicals relative to pharmaceuticals (figure 1–1) is supportive of this proposition.

Some further factors must be considered, however, to gain insight from these findings into the effects of the VFC program on R&D investments. In particular, to determine whether the VFC program will significantly affect research intensities through its effect on expected returns, one needs to know how the program will change firm expectations concerning the prices and revenues realized by future vaccine introductions.

One approach in this regard is to assume that firms will base their expectations about new vaccines on what happens to the sales revenues and margins of established children's vaccines. If this is the case, the effect of increasing government purchases under the VFC program on vaccine R&D would be highly negative. In this regard, Mercer Management has estimated that if government purchases of childhood vaccines increase to 78 percent of the total market from the 50 percent levels prevalent in recent years, sales of these vaccines would decline by $175 million. This represents a 24 percent decline in total market revenues. Furthermore, unit margins would be expected to exhibit a greater percentage decline than would sales revenues, since reductions in costs are likely to be proportionately less than the reductions in sales revenues. The negative effect on expected returns is large.

The price discounts to the VFC program for new vaccines, of course, are not formally tied to those that prevail on established vaccines. The firm must negotiate a price with the CDC on a case-by-case basis for each new vaccine that is covered by the VFC program. The varicella vaccine (Varivax) provides the first example of this process. For VFC purchases of Varivax, the government and Merck agreed to an 18 percent discount relative to the private sector price in its initial one-year contract.[5] This is a relatively modest discount compared with those that now prevail for older, established vaccines. If this type of discount were to prevail over subsequent contract periods and become the norm for new vaccines, it could help to ameliorate concerns about the effects of further expansion in the VFC program on the returns to vaccine R&D investment.[6] Firms with products in the pipeline, however, would still be subject to uncertainty about changes in the purchasing policies of future administrations.

Since the level of cash flow affects the marginal cost of funds (figure 3–2, panel A), further expansion of VFC purchases will also affect R&D investments through this supply side of the market. It is instructive to consider the magnitude of this effect. Relying on our earlier work covering 1962–1975 and the results reported here covering 1974–1989, it seems reasonable to take about 25 percent of cash flows as the effect on R&D investment. Hence, if increasing public purchases to 78 percent of the U.S. market under VFC results in a reduction in cash flow of $90 million–$120 million per year, it would be reasonable to translate this into reduced annual R&D investments of $22.5 million–$30 million using the 25 percent cash flow effect on R&D.[7]

A relevant issue is how much of this reduction in R&D would occur in pediatric vaccines. As noted, any VFC-induced reduction in cash flow results in an increase in the marginal cost of funds (figure 3–2, panel A). The extent to which the increased cost of funds will spill over to other divisions of the firm depends on the organizational structure of the firm. Under the traditional centralized control model of the firm, investment budgets are allocated centrally in accordance with the expected returns of each division. Under this organizational approach, the R&D reductions across areas will depend on the relative shape of the MRR curves in different divisions (figure 3–2, panel

A). In particular, those divisions with the most elastic MRR curves would suffer the biggest decreases in R&D expenditures.

A more decentralized model of firm organizational structure, however, would predict that the significant R&D cutbacks would occur in vaccines. Under this alternative model of organizational behavior, divisions are managed as quasi-independent profit centers. In this situation, each division has some priority claim on cash flows that it generates. The central management still has final authority over investment allocation decisions, but their focus is on emerging investment areas and adjustments for transitory changes occurring within particular divisions. Under this model, reductions in cash flow that are expected to be permanent in nature would primarily affect the claims of the vaccine division for future investment funds.

In summary, although one cannot precisely quantify reductions that would occur in R&D expenditures, there are strong reasons to believe that they will be significant in nature. Our empirical analysis in table 4–1 indicates that R&D expenditures for pharmaceutical firms are highly sensitive to both expected returns and cash flows. If the government were to displace most of the private market in vaccines and to retain its traditional, heavily discounted purchasing policies, the effect on cash flow and expected returns would be very negative for the reasons presented above. Furthermore, the added uncertainty for business decisions would be a heavy burden for R&D investments in vaccines that can span a decade or more before positive cash flows are earned.

Vaccine R&D of Biotech Firms

One potential qualification concerns the sample of firms used for estimates—that is, established pharmaceutical companies—and the fact that a large amount of R&D for vaccines is now carried out by small biotech firms. Two points can be made in this regard. First, much of the financing of new biotech firms derives from the established pharmaceutical firms. For example, American Home Products has pledged at least $100 million to underwrite DNA vaccine research by the small biotech firm Apollon, and Merck has a similar pledge to another small firm, Vical.[8] Second, as we noted earlier, most biotech firms are small, with little cash flow, and they rely heavily on venture capital. In congressional testimony, chief executive officers of biotech firms state that they are therefore "exquisitely sensitive" to signals from Washington (like the VFC program). Hence, one might reasonably conclude that biotech R&D expenditures will react more negatively than will the R&D expenditures of vaccine divisions of the established pharmaceutical companies.

Biotech firms developing new pediatric vaccines must compete with other entrepreneurial ventures for scarce capital. Lance Gordon, CEO of OraVax, indicates that in order to obtain venture capital, a new project must have the ability to generate a 25–35 percent annual rate of return (based on a cash-flow analysis discounted for time to market).[9] The hurdle rate is set this high because of the high risks surrounding discovery-stage R&D projects and the availability of competing investment projects capable of earning these returns. In addition, investors must see a viable exit strategy on getting their money out of the company—that is, through an initial public offering, a merger, or a corporate partnership with an established company. The ability to attract a corporate partner plays a crucial role for biotech firms not only as a source of additional funding, but also as a means of validating the technology.

The potential of the VFC program to displace most of the private market for vaccines creates basic uncertainty in the minds of venture capitalists concerning whether new pediatric vaccines that are technologically successful can earn an acceptable rate of return. There are few if any cases of venture capitalists supporting industries subject to government-controlled pricing. In addition, by making corporate partnership arrangements more problematic, it makes it difficult for biotech firms with initial funding for vaccine R&D to follow through to the next stages of development. At present, there is an abundance of promising alternative venture capital projects for adult vaccines, other medical therapies, and entrepreneurial projects outside the health care system that are not subject to government pricing control. The VFC program imposes a substantial burden of additional perceived risk on pediatric vaccine R&D projects on top of all the other expected risks associated with discovering and developing a new therapeutic agent.

5

Conclusions and Policy Issues

The traditional role for government in vaccines has been the provision of free vaccination for the poor and near poor and the prevention of infectious diseases through vaccination requirements. The VFC program supports these basic goals but also has the potential to expand vastly the public market for pediatric vaccines. In this regard, the legislation offers incentives for the states to provide vaccines free of charge on a universal basis to all residents. The purported objective is to remove price as a barrier to vaccination. As the GAO and other investigators have pointed out, however, price is not currently a major barrier to vaccination in the United States. Low vaccination rates are more related to such factors as parental incentives, parental education, and poorly functioning medical delivery systems.

In an era when both the government and private sectors are searching for flexible, cost-effective options in health care, the federal encouragement of more universal-purchase states under the VFC program is a very cost-ineffective policy intervention. This kind of expansion would in effect subsidize many wealthy families that now have vaccine coverage through the private market and produce at best incremental increases in vaccination rates at high public cost. The objectives of higher vaccination rates can be better achieved by instituting targeted programs that address the primary causes of low vaccinations.

Beyond these traditional policy considerations, a major finding of the current study is that significantly expanding the government sector in pediatric vaccines will also lead to unintended adverse consequences with respect to the search for new vaccines. R&D projects for new vaccines and pharmaceuticals are very risky activities that involve large out-of-pocket investment outlays over long time spans. A firm contemplating investing millions of dollars annually over a decade or more for a new pediatric vaccine must make these decisions on expectations about future market conditions. The prospect of an expanding government market replacing existing private market coverage at controlled prices lowers the expected returns on new pediatric vaccines. Increasing the government share of existing pediatric vaccines also reduces the cash flows available to finance R&D for new vaccines. Our empirical analysis indicates that the R&D investments for pharmaceuticals and vaccines have been highly sensitive to both these factors.

Eliminating most of the private market for vaccines and substituting government purchases at lower prices sends the message to R&D investors that tomorrow's pediatric vaccine breakthroughs are to be valued less than other medical breakthroughs. As a consequence, one would expect R&D resources to shift to substitute projects such as adult vaccines, pharmaceuticals, and other investment alternatives. The greatest negative effect would be on long-term discovery research for vaccines. This research is the riskiest and furthest away from commercial introduction. Discovery research in vaccines has been pursued vigorously in recent years by several smaller biotech firms. These firms are especially vulnerable to an increased government share in this market.

A reduction in R&D investment for new vaccines would be a very unfortunate outcome because the scientific opportunities in this area have proliferated in the past decade. New research techniques associated with biotechnology and related fields have played a major role in enhancing the search for new vaccines. There are many important vaccines currently in the research and development pipeline, including safer versions of existing vaccines and new vaccines for diseases such as rotavirus, otitis media, respiratory syncytial virus, herpes, and many others.[1] It is ironic that a government program designed to advance children's health care could ultimately produce unintended consequences that would lead to fewer opportunities for improved health care in future periods.

Appendix

In table A–1 we present the linear regression coefficient estimates for four cases. Equations (1) and (3) cover the entire period, 1974–1989. Equations (2) and (4) cover the 1980s only. The first two equations employ the *Imarg* variable to capture the demand effect; the last two equations use *Newsal* to proxy the demand effect. The specifications of the variables are given at the bottom of the table.

Turning to table A–2, a different specification is used. In the table, an interaction variable is introduced—*CashPC*—which is simply the product of *Cashfl* and *Pcpharm*. This specification allows for the effect of *Cashfl* on the R&D intensity to vary with *Pcpharm*. Similarly, we introduce interaction variables for the two demand effect variables—*Imarg* and *Newsal*.

These specifications yield quite similar results regarding the effect of *Cashfl* and the demand variables, *Imarg* and *Newsal*. Table A–3 compares the results from all regressions. The equations that include the interaction variables are evaluated at the mean value of *Pcpharm*—or 54 percent. Table A–4 provides the sample means for all the variables.

TABLE A–1
LINEAR REGRESSIONS EXPLAINING
R&D TO SALES RATIO FOR ELEVEN FIRMS

Equation	*1*[a]	*2*[b]	*3*[a]	*4*[b]
Intercept	–0.20 (–7.00)	–0.17 (–4.75)	–0.06 (–8.04)	–0.07 (–4.02)
Imarg	0.74 (6.58)	0.62 (4.46)		
Newsal			0.17 (7.95)	0.19 (3.55)
Cashfl	0.27 (9.88)	0.29 (8.01)	0.28 (11.05)	0.31 (8.40)
Pcpharm	0.05 (4.57)	0.05 (3.65)	0.04 (4.58)	0.04 (3.25)
Rsq/F	0.71/140.8	0.72/91.6	0.74/159.2	0.70/84.2
N	176	110	176	110

NOTES:

Imarg = Industry margin, weighted average pre-tax profits as percent of sales taken from data for pharmaceutical divisions of eleven major health-oriented firms.

Newsal = Average new product sales (first three years) for industry NCEs introduced in years 0, –1, –2, –3, and –4, all divided by real R&D expenditures in year –2.

Cashfl = Cash flow for firm divided by sales, where cash flow = profits after taxes, plus depreciation, plus R&D costs, divided by sales, all lagged by two years.

Pcpharm = Percentage of total firm sales accounted for by pharmaceutical sales.

a. 1974–1989.

b. 1980–1989.

SOURCE: Authors.

TABLE A–2
LINEAR REGRESSIONS EXPLAINING R&D TO SALES RATIO FOR ELEVEN FIRMS, USING INTERACTION VARIABLES, 1974–1989

Equation	*1*	*2*	*3*	*4*
Intercept	–0.17 (–6.37)	–0.18 (–6.64)	–0.03 (–4.65)	–0.03 (–4.56)
Imarg	0.64 (5.87)	0.76 (6.96)		
Newsal			0.08 (3.11)	0.17 (8.36)
Cashfl	0.27 (9.84)	0.11 (2.16)	0.28 (11.21)	0.12 (2.71)
CashPC		0.27 (5.64)		0.26 (5.72)
ImargPC	0.19 (4.65)			
NewsalPC			0.17 (4.81)	
Rsq/F	0.71/ 141.5	0.73/ 152.0	0.74/ 161.7	0.75/ 172.4
N	176	176	176	176

NOTES:

CashPC = Percentage of total firm sales accounted for by pharmaceutical sales multiplied by *Cashfl*.

ImargPC = Percentage of total firms' sales accounted for by pharmaceutical sales multiplied by *Imarg*.

NewsalPC = Percentage of total firms' sales accounted for by pharmaceutical sales multiplied by *Newsal*.

SOURCE: Authors.

TABLE A–3
SUMMARY OF DEMAND AND CASH FLOW EFFECTS

Variable	*Coefficients*	*Location of Equation*
Imarg	0.74	Table A–1, eq 1
	0.62	Table A–1, eq 2
	0.76	Table A–2, eq 2
	0.74	Table A–2, eq 1
Newsal	0.17	Table A–1, eq 3
	0.19	Table A–1, eq 4
	0.17	Table A–2, eq 4
	0.17	Table A–2, eq 3
Cashfl	0.27	Table A–1, eq 1
	0.29	Table A–1, eq 2
	0.28	Table A–1, eq 3
	0.31	Table A–1, eq 4
	0.27	Table A–2, eq 1
	0.28	Table A–2, eq 3
	0.25	Table A–2, eq 2
	0.26	Table A–2, eq 4

NOTE: All variables are evaluated at *Pcpharm* = 0.54, sample mean, where *Pcpharm* is the percentage of total firm sales accounted for by pharmaceutical sales.
SOURCE: Authors.

TABLE A–4
MEANS OF VARIABLES

Variables	*1974–1989*	*1980–1989*
R&D /Sales	0.074	0.083
Imarg	0.255	0.259
Newsal	0.266	0.305
Cashfl	0.212	0.219
Pcpharm	0.536	0.536

SOURCE: Authors.

Notes

Chapter 1: The U.S. Vaccine Industry

1. Much of the information in this section is drawn from Mercer Management Consulting's June 1995 report for the Department of Health and Human Services, *Report on the United States Vaccine Industry*, and from the 1993 Institute of Medicine report, Violaine S. Mitchell, Nalini M. Philipose, and Jay P. Sanford, eds., *The Children's Vaccine Initiative.*

2. In a 1996 presentation to Wall Street, J. Stephenne of SmithKline Beecham estimated that the size of the world vaccine market in 1995 was $3.3 billion.

3. While foreign entry into the U.S. vaccine market has been insignificant because of stringent licensing requirements, there have been a number of alliances in recent years outside the United States in the form of joint ventures and licensing agreements among the major firms. For a discussion of this issue, see David C. Mowery and Violaine Mitchell, "An Assessment of the Feasibility and Market Impact of Expanded Foreign Firm Participation," in Mark Pauly et al., eds., *Supplying Vaccines: An Economic Analysis of Critical Issues* (Amsterdam: IOS Press, 1996), pp. 201–6.

4. Between 1993 and 1996 the government switched to purchasing DTP in combination with the Hib vaccines (DTP/Hib), as well as the new acellular pertussis formulation of this vaccine (DTaP). It stopped purchasing DTP in August 1996.

5. In a telephone conversation on April 2, 1997, Bob Snyder at the CDC indicated that based on the data compiled to date, government purchases of the pediatric vaccines in the program were estimated to account for 65 to 70 percent of the U.S. mar-

ket for these vaccines in 1996. This compares with a 58 percent government share in 1995 and 50 percent share in the 1992–1993 period.

6. Statement of Mercer Management Consulting before the Subcommittee on Health and the Environment of the House Committee on Commerce, June 15, 1995.

7. Much of the material in this section is based on U.S. General Accounting Office, *Vaccines for Children: Re-examination of Program Goals and Implementation Needed to Ensure Vaccination*, GAO/PEMD-95-22 (Washington, D.C., June 1995).

8. The universal purchase states in 1994 were Alaska, Connecticut, Idaho, Maine, Massachusetts, New Hampshire, North Carolina, Rhode Island, South Dakota, Vermont, Washington, and Wyoming.

9. *New York Times*, February 2, 1993.

10. See Robert M. Goldberg, *The Vaccines for Children Program*, Washington, D.C.: AEI Press, 1995, p. 8.

11. GAO Report, *Vaccines for Children*, Executive Summary, chapter 3: "Results in Brief," p. 3.

12. The three additional universal purchase states are Nevada, New Mexico, and North Dakota. Furthermore, the CDC indicated that by the end of 1996, fifteen other states provided publicly purchased vaccines to all health providers for the underinsured population. In these quasi-universal purchase states, children who have health insurance that does not cover immunizations may obtain free vaccines from any provider rather than having to go to a public health clinic. The fifteen states in this category are Arizona, Florida, Georgia, Hawaii, Illinois, Kentucky, Maryland, Michigan, Minnesota, Missouri, Montana, New York, Oklahoma, South Carolina, and Texas.

13. See the GAO Report, *Vaccines for Children*, chapter 4: "Promising Options," for a discussion of some of these studies and public policy programs specifically designed to address these barriers.

14. Since 1993, two of the domestic pediatric vaccine producers (Lederle and Wyeth) have been owned by a single firm as a result of a merger. At the same time, there are pending applica-

tions for entry into the industry of two biotech firms, Chiron and North American Vaccine, and there are other potential entrants as a result of the renaissance in vaccine R&D discussed below.

15. Institute of Medicine, *Vaccine Supply and Innovation* (Washington, D.C.: National Academy Press, 1985).

16. Burton A. Weisbrod, "Costs and Benefits of Medical Research: A Case Study of Poliomyelitis," *Journal of Political Economy,* vol. 79 (1971), pp. 527–44.

17. Chester A. Robinson and Stephen J. Sepe, "Immunization Policies for the 1990s and Beyond," in Mark Pauly et al., eds., *Supplying Vaccines: An Economic Analysis of Critical Issues* (Amsterdam: IOS Press, 1996), pp. 34–35. Tracy A. Lieu et al., "Cost Effectiveness of a Routine Varicella Vaccination Program for U.S. Children," *JAMA,* February 2, 1994, vol. 271, pp. 375–81.

18. Joseph Weber, "Turning Genes into Vaccines," *Business Week,* June 24, 1996, pp. 154–56.

19. Biologicals in this case comprise bacterial and virus vaccines, antigens, antitoxins, toxoids, serums, plasmas, and other blood derivatives for human use.

20. National Institutes of Health, *The Jordan Report, Accelerated Development of Vaccines 1996,* Bethesda, Maryland, 1996.

21. Biotechnology Medicines in Development 1996 Survey, PhRMA, Washington, D.C., June 1996.

22. Joseph Weber, "Turning Genes into Vaccines," *Business Week,* June 24, 1996, pp. 154–56.

23. Statement of J. Leighton Read before the Subcommittee on Health and the Environment of the House Committee on Commerce, June 15, 1995.

Chapter 2: Economics of Vaccine Innovation

1. H. Grabowski and J. Vernon, "Returns to R&D on New Drug Introductions in the 1980s," *Journal of Health Economics,* vol. 13, November 1994, pp. 383–406.

2. Merrile Sing and Mary Kaye Willian, "Supplying Vaccines: An Overview of the Context," in Mark Pauly et al., *Supplying Vaccines,* p. 66.

3. *Federal Register,* May 14, 1996, p. 24, 228.

4. Joseph A. DiMasi, Ronald W. Hansen, Henry G. Grabowski, and Louis Lasagna, "Cost of Innovation in the Pharmaceutical Industry," *Journal of Health Economics,* vol. 10, 1991, pp. 107–42.

5. If one updates this number for inflation using the CPI, the R&D costs would now be over $300 million. There is indication, however, that R&D costs have been increasing faster than inflation based on aggregate trends in R&D expenditures, INDs, and NCEs. The Center for the Study of Drug Development is undertaking a new study that will update its earlier analysis.

6. Carolyn Hardegree, William Stevens, and Elaine Esber, "The Licensing Process," unpublished paper presented to the National Vaccine Advisory Committee, December 19, 1989.

7. Joseph A. DiMasi, Ronald W. Hansen, Henry G. Grabowski, and Louis Lasagna, "Research and Development Costs for New Drugs by Therapeutic Category: A Study of the U.S. Pharmaceutical Industry," *PharmacoEconomics,* vol. 7, 1995, pp. 152–69.

8. The mean time for NCE introductions in the 1990s from investigational new drug filing to FDA approval was 8.3 years (8.2 years for 1980s NCE introductions). See Joseph A. DiMasi, "A New Look at United States Drug Development and Approval Times," *American Journal of Therapeutics,* vol. 3, 1996, pp. 1–11.

9. Brigitta Bienz-Tadmor, Patricia A. Di Cerbo, Gilead Tadmor, and Louis Lasagna, "Biopharmaceuticals and Conventional Drugs: Clinical Success Rates," *Bio/Technology,* vol. 10, May 1992, pp. 521–25.

10. M. M. Struck, "Biopharmaceutical R&D Success Rates and Development Times," *Bio/Technology,* vol. 12, July 1994, pp. 674–77.

11. Marilyn E. Gosse, Joseph A. DiMasi, and Toben F. Nelson, "Recombinant Protein and Therapeutic Monoclonal Antibody Drug Development in the United States: 1980–1994," *Clinical Pharmacology and Therapeutics,* vol. 60, December 1996, pp. 608–18.

12. National Institutes of Health, *The Jordan Report, Accelerated Development of Vaccines 1996,* Bethesda, Maryland, 1996, pp. 9–72.

13. Marilyn E. Gosse and Michael Manocchia, "First Biopharmaceuticals Approved in the U.S.: 1980–1994," *Drug Information Journal,* vol. 30, 1996, pp. 991–1001.

14. Violaine S. Mitchell, Nalini M. Philipose, and Jay P. Sanford, eds., *The Children's Vaccine Initiative,* Institute of Medicine (Washington, D.C.: National Academy Press, 1993), p. 114.

15. Ibid., p. 119.

16. Hearings before the Subcommittee on Health and the Environment of the House Committee on Commerce, June 15, 1995.

17. Frederick G. Bader, "Manufacturing Facilities Planning: Impact on Pharmaceutical Competitiveness." Paper presented to Tufts University Workshop on Biotechnology, September 16, 1992.

18. NIS Feasibility Study, "Manufacturing Facility for Diphtheria, Tetanus, and Pertussis Vaccine and Oral Polio Vaccine." Paper prepared for U.S. Agency for International Development by Lederle-Praxis Biologicals, Wayne, New Jersey, October 1993.

19. Ibid, p. I.2.

20. Mitchell et al., *The Children's Vaccine Initiative,* p. 85.

21. Ibid, p. 101.

22. Mercer Management Consulting, *Report on the United States Vaccine Industry,* June 1995.

23. Henry Grabowski and John Vernon, "Longer Patents for Increased Generic Competition: The Waxman-Hatch Act after One Decade," *PharmacoEconomics,* vol. 10, Suppl. 2, 1996, pp. 110–23.

24. Mercer Report, p.27.

25. Mitchell et al., *The Children's Vaccine Initiative,* p.99.

26. Mercer Report, p. 31.

27. Testimony of R. Gordon Douglas, Jr., President, Merck Vaccine Division, before Senate Committee on Finance, May 6, 1993.

28. J. Leighton Read, Chairman and CEO, Aviron, Inc., Statement before the House Subcommittee on Health and the Environment of the House Committee on Commerce, June 15, 1995.

Chapter 3: A Conceptual Model

1. See, for example, Steven M. Fazzar, R. Glenn Hubbard, and Bruce C. Petersen, "Financing Constraints and Corporate Investment," *Brookings Papers on Economic Activity,* 1, 1988.

2. Henry Grabowski and John Vernon, "The Determinants of R&D Expenditures in the Pharmaceutical Industry," in Robert Helms, ed., *Drugs and Health* (Washington, D.C.: AEI Press, 1981).

Chapter 4: An Empirical Analysis

1. Henry Grabowski and John Vernon, "The Determinants of R&D Expenditures in the Pharmaceutical Industry," in Robert Helms, ed., *Drugs and Health* (Washington, D.C.: AEI Press 1981).

2. The eleven firms are Abbott, American Home Products, Bristol Myers, Johnson & Johnson, Lilly, Merck, Pfizer, Schering Plough, Syntex, Upjohn, and Warner-Lambert.

3. The late 1970s and early 1980s witnessed some major new drugs that were "designed" to fit receptor sites—most notably Tagamet. All firms were aware of the shift to rational drug design. Hence, in our view, the increased expectations for R&D were more linked to industry-wide developments than to individual firm successes.

4. The relationship between R&D and cash flow is in fact expected to be a distributed lag involving several periods. Rather than using a fully distributed lag specification, we use a two-year lag to capture this relationship. Our earlier work indicated that little was gained statistically by adding several lag terms versus the two-year lag specification.

5. The direct price for Varivax in the initial contract was $39.94 per dose, whereas the government contract price was $32.70 per dose for orders of fewer than 500 doses and $32.40 per dose for orders in excess of 500 doses. FDC Reports, "The Pink Sheet," May 20, 1996, pp. T & G 5.

6. A historical example, however, shows a very different life cycle pattern. The conjugated Hib vaccine initially was purchased under government contract in 1988 at a discount of 20 percent to the catalog price. In the second year of the contract, the government discount increased to 56 percent, and by 1993 it had grown to 65 percent. Pauly et al., *Supplying Vaccines,* p. 74.

7. This estimate of the effects of VFC on cash flows is from Mercer Management Consulting, based on their analysis for HHS.

Statement of Mercer Management Consulting before the Subcommittee on Health and the Environment of the House Committee on Commerce, June 15, 1995.

8. *Business Week,* June 24, 1996, p. 154.

9. Hearings before the Subcommittee on Health and the Environment, June 15, 1995.

Chapter 5: Conclusions and Policy Issues

1. National Institutes of Health, *The Jordan Report, Accelerated Development of Vaccines 1996,* Bethesda, Maryland, 1996.

Index

About the Authors

HENRY G. GRABOWSKI is professor of economics and director of the Program in Pharmaceuticals and Health Economics at Duke University. He has also been a research associate at the National Bureau of Economic Research and a visiting scholar in the Office of Research of the Health Care Financing Administration. His writing on the economics of innovation and government regulation of business includes *The Regulation of Pharmaceuticals: Balancing the Benefits and Risks,* cowritten with John Vernon, and his recent work "The Impact of Cost-Effectiveness on Public and Private Policies in Health Care: An International Perspective," coedited with Frank Sloan, in *Social Science and Medicine.*

JOHN M. VERNON is professor of economics at Duke University. He also served on the faculties of the University of Bristol and Harvard University. Mr. Vernon was project director at Marketing Science Institute in Cambridge, Massachusetts. His research interests include industrial organization and public policy, the economics of innovation and regulation, and applied microeconomics. He has published numerous books and articles in those areas, including *Economics of Regulation and Antitrust,* coauthored with W. K. Viscusi and J. Harrington.

The American Enterprise Institute for Public Policy Research

Founded in 1943, AEI is a nonpartisan, nonprofit, research and educational organization based in Washington, D. C. The Institute sponsors research, conducts seminars and conferences, and publishes books and periodicals.

AEI's research is carried out under three major programs: Economic Policy Studies; Foreign Policy and Defense Studies; and Social and Political Studies. The resident scholars and fellows listed in these pages are part of a network that also includes ninety adjunct scholars at leading universities throughout the United States and in several foreign countries.

The views expressed in AEI publications are those of the authors and do not necessarily reflect the views of the staff, advisory panels, officers, or trustees.

This book was edited by
Cheryl Weissman
of the American Enterprise Institute.
The index was prepared by Julia Petrakis.
The text was set in New Baskerville.
Electronic Quill set the type,
and Edwards Brothers, Incorporated,
of Lillington, North Carolina,
printed and bound the book,
using permanent acid-free paper.

The AEI Press is the publisher for the American Enterprise Institute for Public Policy Research, 1150 Seventeenth Street, N.W., Washington, D.C. 20036; *Christopher DeMuth,* publisher; *Dana Lane,* director; *Ann Petty,* editor; *Leigh Tripoli,* editor; *Cheryl Weissman,* editor; *Jennifer Lesiak,* production manager.